SURVIVING

TO

Thriving

SURVIVING
TO
Thriving

A Six-Step Blueprint to Narcissistic Abuse Healing and Recovery

Lisa Sonni
Kerry Kerr McAvoy, Ph.D.

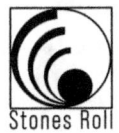

Stones Roll

CONTENT

INTRODUCTION

Lisa's Story

It all started with an instant connection. I remember feeling drawn to him, despite him not being my usual type. His charm, magnetism, and persistence had me feeling special and seen. But as time went on, I couldn't help but notice that something felt off. He was hot and cold, and I struggled to keep up with the constant emotional rollercoaster. It wasn't until years later that I realized what was really happening. The "meant to be" feelings were manufactured, and I was in too deep to notice. I was convinced that his mistreatment of me was due to his childhood trauma, recently discovered addictions and that I could love it out of him.

I was unaware of narcissism in the true sense, and spent my time in the relationship feeling alone, even when he was right beside me. I entered individual psychotherapy hoping for validation and clarity of what I was experiencing and feeling, but instead, I was invalidated. I was diagnosed with anxiety shortly thereafter, and it felt like I was sinking deeper and deeper into the abyss. It took two violent assaults and even more physical abuse for me to realize that I was in an abusive relationship.

It's hard to describe the depth of pain and confusion that comes with narcissistic abuse. It's like being trapped in a never-ending cycle of love and heartbreak, constantly feeling like you're not good enough but always striving to be. For me, it took years to realize what was happening and even longer to fully heal from the trauma.

I found Narctok on TikTok as my relationship spiraled. Strangers online shared their stories, and I felt like they were speaking directly to me. The level of deception I experienced was astounding, but it was also a turning point. I let go and began to heal. As I recovered, I authored an online course and several books on breaking trauma bonds to help others learn and escape their own abusive relationships. Recovery felt impossible at first, but with time and effort, I was able to overcome the emotional obstacles that had been eating away at me. This book outlines the steps I took to heal, and I hope it helps others on their journey to recovery.

This book is my way of paying it forward. It's a guide to help others who have suffered from narcissistic abuse, to show them that they're not alone and that recovery is possible. It's a reminder that no matter how dark things may seem, there is always hope for a brighter tomorrow.

Kerry's Story

Dazed and scared, I arrived in the United States empty-handed except for two large suitcases. My oldest son, barely 28 years old, was sick with leukemia and lay inches from death. Through I'd returned to the States with my new husband, his disinterested look told me all I needed to know. Our recent marriage, which had just celebrated its second anniversary, was ending.

Two weeks later, my soon-to-be ex walked out. That was the last of my worries, though since I was facing the possibility of losing a kid. The evenings and nights alone in a strange, new town were the worst; in the night's pitch-blackness fear would threatened to smother me and tears would drip down the sides of my cheeks as I cried myself to sleep, but I'd pull myself together each day to sit by my oldest's hospital bed. Though I lacked the words to describe what I'd survived during the last relationship, I couldn't stop talking about it.

Unfamiliar with narcissistic abuse despite my training and work experience as a psychologist, I joined an online support group for separated and divorced women of sex addicts. Three hours a week, I listened to these women describe abuse and mistreatment. Meanwhile, I struggled to make sense of what I'd survived. I had no idea I was suffering from chronic and persistent cognitive dissonance and was in the throes of breaking a trauma bond. To cope, I began to pour my story out onto the page, at first with an intense need to tattle, then later with a burning desire to save others from this experiencing this terrible trauma.

As the book, *Love You More: The Harrowing Tale of Lies, Sex Addiction, & Double Cross* neared completion, I stumbled across Narctok on TikTok and met Lisa Sonni along with several other groundbreaking creators. Slowly I learned the vocabulary of narcissistic abuse, and the pieces began to fit together.

Narcissistic abuse is a horrific attack on a person's selfhood. It erodes an individual's agency, autonomy, and confidence as it distorts their perception of reality and sense of self. But, just like there is a pattern that defines this type of abuse, there is also a blueprint for its healing. The steps outlined in this workbook are what saved me and, undoubtfully, Lisa as well. We give it to you with our hopes for your full recovery. None of us ever asked to have our identities battered and bruised by toxic love, but healing is possible. I've found it, and you can find it too.

Overview of the Workbook

Welcome to *Surviving To Thriving: A Six-Step Blueprint to Narcissistic Abuse Recovery and Healing*. This empowering guide was crafted with love and empathy by two survivors of narcissistic abuse, a coach and a psychologist, who have not only walked the walk, but have also healed and now dedicate their lives to helping others do the same. Inside these pages, you'll find practical steps, activities, and coping tools specifically designed to help you overcome the six biggest obstacles survivors face: Letting Go of Potential, Resolving Cognitive Dissonance, Beating the Guilt, Overcoming Fear, Mastering Boundaries, and Improving Self-Worth.

Our mission is to help you transform your pain into newfound strength and resilience so that you can move forward confidently and courageously. We believe in you, and together, we will guide you on your journey from *surviving* to *thriving*. Pay attention to your reactions, thoughts, relationship patterns and dreams while you work through these obstacles.

Surviving To Thriving is not just a guide, but a workbook filled with interactive activities, reflective questions, and writing prompts designed to inspire deep self-exploration to aid emotional healing. To fully benefit from this book, we encourage you to take your time with each step, write down your thoughts and feelings, and engage wholeheartedly in the activities presented. Welcome to your first step towards healing and reclaiming your life.

Letting Go of Potential

If you've survived a relationship with a narcissist, you are no stranger to the pain and confusion that occur within these partnerships. Narcissists pretend to be someone they are not, and victims fall in love with the fake persona, the mask. Most likely, you were promised an amazing life. Narcissists used future faking to sell the possibility of an idealized dream that never materializes.

Unsurprisingly, survivors of narcissistic abuse find it difficult to let go of this seemingly perfect potential. To do so requires each of us to focus on living in reality. Reclaiming your power after abuse is a process that starts with recognizing it is time to leave an unhealthy situation and ends with mastering post-trauma emotions. Each step helps to build internal strength while bringing you closer to regaining self-worth and confidence.

> *Closure happens right after you accept that letting go and moving on is more important than projecting a fantasy of how the relationship could have been.*

Sylvester McNutt

LETTING GO OF POTENTIAL

When leaving a narcissistic relationship, it is common to feel like you were never known--that your most authentic self was overlooked. Narcissists avoid risking vulnerability by faking their way through a relationship. Instead, they use false promises and emotional avoidance, leaving you alone and empty.

The first step to moving on is understanding that a narcissistic relationship is built on pretenses. Your partner's words of love and affirmation were disingenuous; they said what they thought you wanted to hear. Their interest was not in getting to know you but making you cooperative and compliant.

It is important to remember that a narcissist will never change. They will never see you as an equal; in their minds, you are a means to an end. Holding onto the potential of what could have been only leaves you frustrated and disappointed. Instead, let go of that potential and focus on reality.

You are worthy of love and respect. You deserve to be with someone who sees you for who you are and loves you unconditionally. Someone willing to work through the tough times rather than using them as an opportunity to hurt and control you. Healing requires learning how to settle for nothing less than what you deserve.

Mastering these six steps will help you let go of the potential.

1. Recognize when it is time to leave.
2. Identify your limiting beliefs.
3. Change your story.
4. Stop blaming yourself.
5. Forgive yourself.
6. Master your emotions.

LETTING GO OF POTENTIAL

You're already letting go just by being here....

1. Recognize When It's Time To Let Go

When did you first know something was off?

_____

_____

_____

Do (or did) the pleasurable moments outweigh the painful ones in this relationship ? Why or why not?

_____

_____

_____

In what way(s) have you been future faked?

_____

_____

_____

_____

Is or was that future ever attainable based on their actions?

_____

_____

_____

_____

2. Identify Your Self-Limiting Beliefs

Limiting Beliefs are negative self-perceptions that live in our conscious and unconscious mind. They are rooted in past experiences, feedback from others, our family and friends' values and beliefs, and even messages we get from the media (or social media).

List a few of your limiting beliefs.

_____

_____

_____

_____

It is helpful to replace our limiting beliefs with empowering ones.

What if something bad happens?

⬇

What if this is the best thing to ever happen to me?

Take two of your limiting beliefs and reframe them

First

_____

Limiting

⬇

_____

Empowering

Second

_____

Limiting

⬇

_____

Empowering

3. Change Your Story

We all create a story. It is what you tell yourself based on your limiting beliefs.

"Of course they got angry a lot. I nagged them all the time."

vs.

"I tolerated their anger because I didn't know how to safely stand up for myself."

What story have you created to justify your limiting beliefs?

_____

_____

_____

_____

What assumptions are you making and what are you excusing?

_____

_____

_____

_____

Write a new story that aligns better with your true self.

_____

_____

_____

_____

_____

_____

4. Stop Blaming Yourself

Acknowledging that you could have done things differently is critical in understanding how your decisions affected the outcome. This process helps to identify troublesome themes and patterns that may need changing as well as which parts are outside your control.

What have you blamed yourself for that is beyond your control?

_____

_____

_____

_____

How has self-blame impacted your healing? What purpose does self-blame serve?

_____

_____

_____

_____

Self-compassion is when you see yourself — your actions and inactions, strengths and weaknesses — from a larger non-judgmental context. What can you say to yourself that demonstrates self-compassion?

_____

_____

_____

_____

_____

_____

6. Master Your Emotions

One of the most powerful steps you can take on your healing journey is to learn how to manage and reframe your emotions. Understanding you have survived a terrible emotional rollercoaster will give you the power to cultivate more positive, empowering emotions instead of getting stuck in a cycle of overwhelming negative ones.

Which emotions regarding this relationship are most overwhelming for you.

_____

_____

_____

_____

When you think about "letting go of the relationship's potential," what does that mean? How does doing that feel?

_____

_____

_____

_____

Exercise

Let's practice being in the present. For the next 5 minutes, focus on your breathing. Feel the air, feel your breath, feel your chest rising and setting.

What can you control in your life now?

_____

_____

_____

What can you NOT control about your current situation?

_____

_____

_____

Exercise

Bilateral stimulation is the use of alternating right and left stimulation. The next time you are upset or anxious, take a small object, such as a tennis ball, wireless headphones case, or lip gloss, and toss it from your left to right hand. Doing this has a relaxing effect. Try using it for the next six to eight weeks. If used consistently, you may find a significant reduction in your anxiety.

What emotions are the most unbearable or overwhelming? Describe what is challenging about each one.

_____

_____

_____

Identify the limiting belief contained in the description of each emotion. Now reframe each with an empowering statement.

_____

_____

_____

Notes

_____

_____

_____

_____

_____

_____

_____

_____

_____

_____

_____

_____

_____

_____

_____

_____

_____

_____

_____

_____

_____

_____

Sonni & McAvoy

Resolving Cognitive Dissonance

Cognitive dissonance often complicates recovery from an abusive relationship. Toxic people tend to create a lot of drama and chaos, which obscures the truth. There is what you thought you knew about your partner and what actually happened. Intense confusion, or cognitive dissonance, occurs when what you believe to be real does not align with what you have experienced. You are left wondering if the person you love is fundamentally good but does terrible things or if they are fundamentally bad yet occasionally does good things. This disparity creates two realities, living with the good person while simultaneously surviving the scary one. As difficult as it can be to reconcile these conflicting truths, cognitive dissonance can be resolved. Let's look at how this process works.

The first step to resolving the inner conflict is to recognize that it exists. Next, identify why you stayed in the relationship and what factors helped to keep you in it. And finally, to accept your reality for what it is now rather than focusing on what could or should have been.

You'll never be able to create the right reality if you're not willing to let the wrong reality go.

Lolly Daskal

COGNITIVE DISSONANCE

Causes of Cognitive Dissonance

Cognitive dissonance is the mental confusion caused by holding two conflicting beliefs, values, or attitudes. Our mind seeks consistency between what we think to be true and what we have actually experienced. When misalignment occurs, feelings of unease or distress arise. (Is my abuser good or bad?)

Forced Compliance Behavior

When someone is forced to do something they really don't want to do, dissonance is created between their cognition (I didn't want to do this) and their behavior (I did it).

In what way(s) did this happen to you?

_____

_____

_____

_____

Decision Making

All life-altering decisions come with positive and negative consequences. For example, whatever we decide about a relationship outcome, we will lose certain benefits while gaining others.

So what are the possible negative and positive effects of leaving your toxic relationship?

_____

_____

_____

_____

COGNITIVE DISSONANCE

Effort

Cognitive dissonance is created by deception. Upon meeting us, narcissists and other predatory or intimacy-avoidant people build a false persona. We think we have met a highly compatible partner, not realizing our preferences, habits, and history have been mimicked, mirrored, and parroted back to us. Unbeknownst to us, the toxic person has become two people simultaneously: the false identity—our idealized soulmate and the real self—hidden yet lurking. Our intuition senses something is off, leaving us uneasy, yet in the beginning, the new persona usually is quite convincing.

Think back to your initial contact with the toxic person. What initial uneasiness or reservations did you have at the start of this relationship?

_____

_____

_____

_____

How were those concerns addressed? What led you to handle your discomfort this way?

_____

_____

_____

_____

"If a person finds themselves in a situation where they have to do something that they don't agree with, they'll experience discomfort. Since they can't escape the action, they attempt to re-establish their reasons for doing it in a way that makes the action acceptable."

Allaya Cooks-Campbell

Your Dual Reality

At some point, the false persona slipped, usually after a significant commitment, and you glimpsed the real person. In shock, you began to question if you knew your partner's character. Your partner, however, covered the reveal through denial, lying, and gaslighting, causing you to doubt yourself. So now you have created a simultaneous internalized dual reality of this person: the good guy/woman and the bad one.

Describe the character traits of the 'good' version of them. (See the list of character traits on page 22.)

_____

_____

_____

How did you behave and feel around this version?

_____

_____

_____

How did you assess which version you were interacting with?

_____

_____

_____

How did you react and behave as a result of this? Describe your feelings & actions.

_____

_____

_____

Describe the character traits of the 'bad' version of them

_____

_____

_____

_____

How did you behave and feel around this version?

_____

_____

_____

_____

How did you assess which version you were interacting with?

_____

_____

_____

_____

How did you react and behave as a result of this? Describe your feelings & actions.

_____

_____

_____

_____

When things do not fit together or make sense, we often resort to denial or compartmentalizing the incongruency to explain it away. For example, even though our partner used an insulting name, they still loved us; they were having a bad day, we will tell ourselves. So we make the incompatible details fit so that they make sense, but this process only increases our mental confusion.

Example Character Traits

funny	selfish	generous	trustworthy	creative
adventurous	immature	impatient	wild	intelligent
caring	charming	successful	nice	sneaky
talkative	optimistic	happy	argumentative	humble
jealous	obnoxious	sweet	nosy	cheerful
persuasive	cruel	playful	wise	curious
peaceful	honest	unkind	demanding	polite
jealous	cooperative	clumsy	timid	gentle
gloomy	careful	silly	mysterious	timid
sincere	persistent	open minded	quiet	selfless
selfish	rude	unpredictable	controlling	sensitive
insecure	powerful	volatile	patient	entitled
forgiving	menacing	fair	loyal	determined

Sonni & McAvoy

Resolving Cognitive Dissonance

Change & Challenge Existing Beliefs

Let's challenge some of the beliefs you hold about your partner. What do you know about their childhood, traumas, and behavior? Do you believe they are a good person who sometimes does mean or abusive things?

_____

_____

_____

_____

Let's compare the attributes of a good person. Consider the character traits you have identified already. Does someone who harms a person also care about that individual? How do we show we love another person?

_____

_____

_____

_____

Let's compare what they say to what they do. Does their behavior align with the definition of love? What actions and behaviors do you see? How have you rationalized their abusiveness?

_____

_____

_____

_____

_____

Resolving Cognitive Dissonance

Reducing The Importance of The Beliefs

In addition to the confusion the toxic partner creates with the two personas of the good and bad person, we also have our own reasons for fearing change. For example, you might worry you will never find love again or that being single carries a negative connotation. Perhaps you feel sorry for your toxic partner?

List two of these beliefs.

_____

_____

Belief One: explore the root of this belief & its importance.

Belief Two: explore the root of this belief & its importance.

Resolving Cognitive Dissonance

Tackling The Power of Your Beliefs

Belief One: replace this belief with a true one. How does it make you feel?

Belief Two: replace this belief with a true one. How does it make you feel?

Calming Your Senses Excercise

Reduce anxiety using this technique.

- Identify five things to look at in your surroundings.
- Listen to four sounds around you.
- Identify three things you can feel and touch.
- Find two things you can smell.
- Discover one thing you can taste.

Resolving Cognitive Dissonance

Identify The Confusion

Abuse survivors are left with a lot of questions: Can our partner change? Is this person good or bad? Did they ever love you? Did we ever really know them?

Which question plagues you the most right now?

_____

_____

_____

_____

What about this issue is bothering you?

_____

_____

_____

What would happen if you made a wrong decision regarding this matter?

_____

_____

_____

How have you dealt with similar situations in the past?

_____

_____

_____

What resources could you rely on to help with the possible outcomes?

_____

_____

Resolving Cognitive Dissonance

The Truth

It can be difficult to accept that abuse is a choice, and that exploitative and manipulative people are not suffering from uncontrollable anger or mental illness. Nor are they a product of childhood trauma or poor parenting. Instead, they have strategically decided to exercise power and control over others.

The confusion caused by cognitive dissonance is deliberate as well. Narcissists and other toxic individuals intentionally hide their identities. Victims receive mixed messages of love and loathing and truth and lies, all designed to keep them off-kilter and immobilized. Unable to ascertain what is real, the victim's dependence on the perpetrator grows. When this confusion is combined with violence, psychological manipulation and intimidation, financial control, isolation, or coercion, the victim's ability to escape is eroded.

As the cognitive dissonance worsens, so does the victim's mental state. Chronic deception slowly erodes the victim's self-confidence as growing self-doubt causes confusion and psychological paralysis. The initial concerns they may have had about their partner's goodness or badness have now turned inwards as they question their sanity. Instead of wondering who their partner is or if the relationship is worth saving, they ask what's wrong with themselves for not leaving.

This deceptive process confounds survivors of narcissistic abuse. Why would their abuser sometimes act kind or lovingly and then abruptly change into a cruel, hurtful person? This baffling pattern is called "the cycle of narcissistic abuse," an emotional roller coaster ride that clouds victims from understanding the reality of their situation.

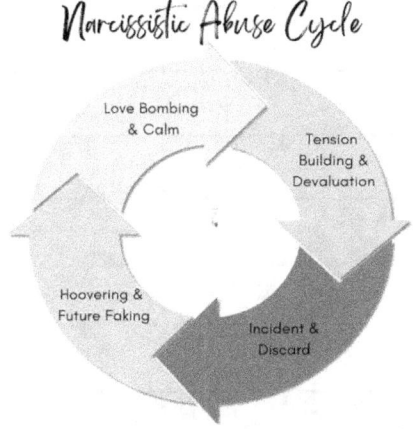

Narcissistic Abuse Cycle

Love Bombing & Calm

Tension Building & Devaluation

Hoovering & Future Faking

Incident & Discard

Notes

Overcoming Fear

Fear can be one of the most powerful emotions that prevent us from leaving. It feeds on a "what-if" mentality. But where do these fears come from? Several different sources interfere with our ability to leave abusive situations. To overcome this obstacle, we will explore a few root causes, learn how to identify early signs of anxiety, and build a coping toolbox.

Fear is a normal reaction to trauma; it is our body's way of telling us that something needs attention. When we experience trauma, such as domestic violence or sexual assault, our primitive mind becomes alert and readies the body to respond protectively. We experience this as fear—fear of leaving our abuser or staying away for too long—and this fear can make it difficult for us to take action, such as deciding to leave an abusive situation. Understanding where these fears come from and identifying the early warning signs helps us arm ourselves with effective management strategies. It gives us an opportunity to design a personalized coping toolbox specific to our needs.

> The scariest moment is always just before you start. After that, things can only get better.
>
> *Stephen King*

OVERCOMING FEAR

Identifying Fears & Limiting Beliefs

What fears do you have about leaving or letting go of this relationship?

_____

_____

_____

_____

Where do these concerns come from? Are they recent or from childhood?

_____

_____

_____

_____

_____

While analyzing your thoughts may not be easy, especially if those thoughts are negative, this practice will provide insight into why you find certain triggers troubling. This understanding will help you address and overcome these fears so that they don't hold you back in the future.

What evidence do you have that supports them being rational or irrational?

_____

_____

_____

_____

_____

_____

_____

OVERCOMING FEAR

Dig Deeper

Using one fear you've identified, recall the event or belief that triggered it. What caused the fear?

_____

_____

_____

_____

What assumptions, thoughts or perceptions are associated with that triggering event or belief?

_____

_____

_____

_____

What were the resulting feelings because of these assumptions?

_____

_____

_____

_____

How have these feelings negatively impacted you or kept you feeling stuck?

_____

_____

_____

Build Your Toolbox

A coping toolbox is a collection of skills, strategies, and resources that help you manage anxiety and other stressors. We will review a variety of techniques. Identifying which methods will work best for you and in which situations is important. Using a combination of tools can build resilience and improve your overall mental health.

Problem-Focused Skills

This process can be as simple as writing out all the possible solutions to your problem, looking into any available resources (such as shelters, legal aid, courses, books, etc.), or asking for advice from someone who has been through a similar experience. Doing any of these steps will provide valuable insight; it breaks the problem into smaller pieces to be more easily managed. Next, we will examine seeking information and breaking down the problem.

Emotion-Focused Skills

These techniques help to manage emotions. Strategies like mindfulness—focusing on being present in the moment—help provide perspective, while positive self-talk boosts confidence, giving the courage to tackle challenges head-on. Activities like journaling or meditation are proven stress reducers—very beneficial when navigating difficult times. We will explore mindfulness and positive self-talk further.

Meaning-Focused Skills

These involve connecting with yourself and others to find meaning beyond what is happening now. Practices, such as gratitude journaling—writing down three things you're thankful for each day, remind you that although this current situation may feel overwhelming, there are still plenty of good things in life to appreciate and anticipate. Connecting with those who have gone through similar experiences is also helpful; not only do they understand what you're going through, but they can offer support and guidance from their healing journey. We will look at few beneficial activities, such as journaling, connecting with others, and using other creative outlets to augment healing.

Build Your Toolbox: Problem-Focused Skills

Seek Information

When faced with anxiety and fear, it's easy to feel overwhelmed and uncertain about what to do. However, it can help to get more information about the situation. Doing this will increase your sense of control and will equip you to handle the problem better. There are various types of resources, such as seeking professional advice, reading books on the topic, researching helpful websites, or joining support groups.

Breakdown The Problem

Anxiety often makes a problem seem larger and more daunting than it is. By breaking down the problem into smaller, more manageable parts, you can approach it more effectively. First, identify the specific aspects causing anxiety and then deconstruct them into smaller steps or tasks. Here's how to do this:

Identify The Problem

First, clearly define the problem. Write down what's causing the anxiety, i.e., When I think of leaving them, I get afraid that I'll be alone for the rest of my life.

Determine The Goal

What do you want to achieve by addressing this problem? Be specific and write down a measurable goal, i.e., I want to leave this abusive relationship for good, knowing it was the right decision.

Build Your Toolbox: Problem-Focused Skills

Brainstorm & Evaluate Solutions

Come up with as many possible solutions as possible. Don't worry if they're good or bad ideas; write them down. For each one, create a list of the pros and cons, then choose the solution most likely to help achieve your goals.

Solution:

Pros	Cons

Solution:

Pros	Cons

Solution:

Pros	Cons

Build Your Toolbox: Problem-Focused Skills

Create a Plan

Break down the chosen solution into small, actionable steps. Create a realistic timeline to complete each step.

Actions

_____

_____

_____

_____

_____

_____

Timeline

_____

_____

_____

_____

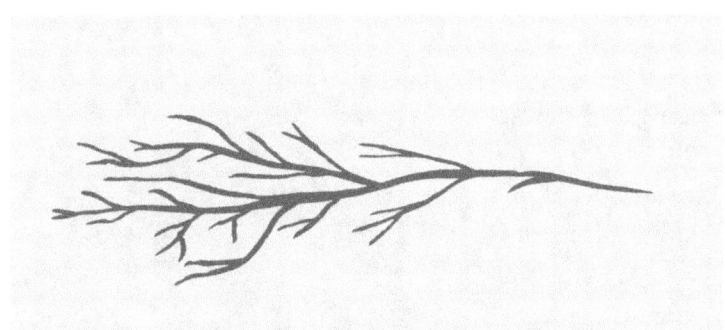

"Give me six hours to chop down a tree and I will spend the
first four sharpening the axe."

Abraham Lincoln

Build Your Toolbox: Emotionally Focused Skills

Mindfulness

Practicing mindfulness techniques, like deep breathing or meditation, can calm the mind and reduce stress. To do this, focus on the present moment, acknowledge your emotions without judgment, and accept them without trying to change them. This technique helps lower anxiety. Here are a few breathing exercises to try.

Acknowledge & Label Your Thoughts

To begin, acknowledge your thoughts are fearful and anxious. Notice your feelings without judgment or trying to push them away. As you continue to observe your inner experience, try labeling them. For example, you might identify a disturbing thought as "fear" or an uneasy one as "anxiety." This process helps create distance between you and your feelings.

Refocus On Your Senses

If other thoughts or concerns start to distract you, recenter by focusing on your senses. Use what you see, hear, and feel around you to bring you back to the present moment. Refer to the Calm Your Senses exercise in the Cognitive Dissonance chapter.

Positive Self-Talk

Reframe negative self-talk into positive affirmations. Try replacing defeatist beliefs with positive ones. Focus on your strengths and what you can control. This will help you feel more empowered and reduce anxiety.

For example:

I am never going to be able to leave and heal.

I don't know how to leave and get over this yet but I'm making progress by learning the tools.

Breathing

Diaphragmatic breathing, also known as belly breathing or deep breathing, is a technique that involves breathing deeply and fully into your belly, rather than shallowly into your chest. This type of breathing helps reduce stress, calms the mind and body, and increases physical relaxation.

Exercise 1

Lie on your back with your knees bent and your feet flat on the floor. Place one hand on your chest and one hand on your belly. Take a slow, deep breath in through your nose, feeling your belly rise and your hand on your belly move outward. Hold your breath for 5 seconds, then slowly exhale through your mouth, feeling your belly fall and your hand on your belly move inward. Repeat for several breaths, focusing on the feeling of your breath in your belly.

Exercise 2

Sit or stand with your back straight and your shoulders relaxed. Place one hand on your chest and one hand on your belly. Take a slow, deep breath in through your nose, feeling your ribcage expand and your hand on your belly move outward. Try to keep your chest still and relaxed. Hold your breath for 5 seconds, then slowly exhale through your mouth, feeling your stomach muscle contract and your hand on your belly move inward. Repeat for several breaths, focusing on the sensation of air moving in and out.

Consider setting a timer several times throughout the day as a reminder to practice these exercises for a few minutes. Or use them whenever you need to settle or calm yourself. With practice, diaphragmatic breathing can become a natural response to stress and anxiety, helping to promote a sense of well-being.

Predicting Triggers

Anxiety can build like a dark cloud of unwelcome thoughts and cast a shadow over your enjoyment of life. It isn't something to ignore or accept as normal, but instead should be considered a vital health concern, an illness we need to combat. Triggers are bound to happen; learning to spot the initial signs can help you get an early jump on addressing them.

Self-Reflection

Reflect on a past experience or two of anxiety or failure. Describe what made you anxious and fearful.

_____

_____

_____

_____

Consider what events or situations led to these experiences. What story are you telling yourself about these situations?

_____

_____

_____

_____

What would happen if you could let go of this fear?

_____

_____

_____

_____

"We must let go of the life we have planned as to accept the one that is waiting for us"

Joseph Campbell

Sonni & McAvoy

Predicting Triggers

Reflect on how you responded to those situations. Were those responses effective? Map out alternative ways to respond.

Situation that caused/s fearful anxiety:

Your past response:

What was the outcome:

Alternative response:

Predicting Triggers

Mindfulness

Make mindfulness techniques, such as meditation or deep breathing, a regular practice. Pay attention to your physical and emotional responses in stressful situations. What happens inside your body? With your breathing?

Observe your triggers and notice any patterns that arise during these situations. Write them down and prepare a plan of action. What will you do when you find yourself feeling anxious or fearful?

Seeking Feedback

Seek feedback from trusted friends, family members, or colleagues. Be careful to exclude those individuals you've identified as toxic or abusive.

When approaching them for feedback, ask questions that will give insight into how others see your behavior during times of stress and anxiety. Ask open-ended questions for a more detailed response, such as: "What have you noticed that I do when I'm feeling overwhelmed?" or "How do I usually respond when I am anxious or fearful?"

Use this feedback to identify areas of difficulty or potential triggers. Then utilize the strategies outlined in this lesson to address them.

By using a combination of self-reflection, mindfulness, and seeking feedback, you will be able to identify anxiety triggers and spot potential signs of trouble before they become overwhelming. This awareness can help you develop effective coping strategies and reduce the impact of anxiety and fear on your well-being.

Notes

Sonni & McAvoy

Beating the Guilt

If you have ever been in an abusive relationship, you are likely familiar with guilt. It is a tool the narcissist uses for dominance. They like to make you think that it is your fault for the relationship's problems, your fault for whatever goes wrong, and your fault for their difficulties and misbehaviors. This terrible feeling of responsibility keeps victims stuck and unable to leave. Like a powerful weapon, guilt gets stirred up to control you. But what if I told you that this feeling is an illusion? That it isn't real?

Guilt can be challenging to shake off. The power of negative stories makes us feel responsible for someone else's suffering—even when we are not. Unfortunately, we tend not to question the logic of this conclusion, making it easy to fall prey to guilt unless something or someone debunks it. It's important to remember that this feeling is not based on reality; it is a misperception used to misdirect you into feeling responsible. This chapter will explore the myth of trauma-related guilt and how to escape its grip.

False guilt is guilt felt at not being what other people feel you ought to be or assume you are.

R. D. Laing

BEATING THE GUILT

Changing Your Emotions

Thoughts and emotions are deeply intertwined, affecting each other in a complex and powerful way. We often believe emotions dictate thoughts and wait for our feelings to change before taking action. However, research shows that when we intentionally change our thoughts, our feelings also change.

Our thoughts are a product of our beliefs, values, and experiences. They provide the lenses through which we view the world and shape our emotions and behaviors. For example, if we tell ourselves, "I didn't do enough to save the relationship," "It's my fault for my family's breakup," or "I stayed too long," we are likely to feel guilty, sad, anxious, or unworthy. Conversely, if we come to the opposite conclusion, such as "I had no choice but to leave because of the abuse," or "I didn't know then what I know now," we are more likely to feel more positive resolve about our decision.

It is difficult to change thoughts because most beliefs are deeply held. However, with practice and persistence, we can learn to question negative or unhelpful thoughts and replace them with more realistic ones. Through the process of reframing situations more positively or considering them from different perspectives, we can begin to question basic assumptions.

Adjust Your Mental State

As a survivor of narcissistic abuse, it can be challenging to shift your focus from the abuser to yourself, but this step is crucial for healing. First, take some time to sit quietly and breathe deeply, focusing on your body's physical sensations. Then, without dwelling on it, acknowledge the pain and hurt you have gone through. Instead, allow yourself to feel your emotions without judgment or criticism.

BEATING THE GUILT

Guilt vs False Guilt

Guilt is a naturally occurring emotion we all experience, but when it comes to narcissistic abuse, distinguishing between real and false guilt can be challenging.

Real guilt is a feeling of remorse or regret that arises when we have done something wrong. False guilt, on the other hand, is feeling responsible for things that are not our fault. Abusers shift blame from themselves to others, making their partners feel liable. Survivors of narcissistic abuse are often made accountable for this person's happiness or behavior, and they may find it difficult to exit the toxic relationship. However, no one is not responsible for someone else's actions or emotions, and leaving an abusive relationship can be a brave and necessary step toward better well-being. False guilt should never keep someone from moving forward.

How did your abuser evoke guilt in your relationship? What words or actions did they use?

_____

_____

_____

_____

Types of Guilt That Commonly Affects Survivors

1. Moral guilt: This type of guilt arises from violating one's own moral code or ethical principles.

2. Shame-based guilt: This type of guilt comes from feeling like one has violated societal norms or expectations.

3. Self-imposed guilt: This type of guilt occurs when a person puts unnecessary pressure on themselves to be perfect or to meet unrealistic expectations.

4. Induced guilt: This type of guilt is imposed by others, either intentionally or unintentionally. Abusers use this intentionally.

Explore The Source

Acknowledge your Feelings

It is important to recognize and validate your feelings of guilt. Understand that it is normal to feel guilty when leaving a relationship, even if the relationship was abusive.

Reflect on Causes

Reflect on the reasons that have made you feel guilty. Do/did you feel like you were abandoning your partner? Do you worry about their well-being? Do you wonder if you made the right decision? Do you question if you stay "too long?"

I feel guilty because:

_____

_____

_____

_____

Your abuser wants you to feel guilty because that negative feeling benefits them. Remember that your guilt does not reflect the effort you've put in.

Describe how you have been manipulated or blamed.

_____

_____

_____

_____

"False guilt is rooted in deception, denial, and dysfunction.
It is directly connected to our destructive and codependent
relationship with a narcissist."

Dana Arcuri

Explore The Truth

Is it possible for you to have an unbiased perspective of the relationship? Can you take a balanced view? Challenge your feelings of guilt by asking if they are based on facts or assumptions. Consider the evidence that supports your decision to leave the relationship. Remember, your compassionate nature most likely has been used against you.

False guilt is an illusion that has nothing to do with what is factual or accurate. It is the fear of disapproval disguised. You have been conditioned to believe you are responsible for your abuser's behavior and emotions, a form of psychological manipulation used by abusers to control victims. This type of guilt damages the victim's self-esteem and sense of self-worth. Your partner wants you to believe that you are the root cause of their suffering when, in fact, they have done it to themselves. Remember, abuse is a choice.

What evidence do you have that suggests you caused their suffering?

_____

_____

_____

_____

It is crucial to challenge the belief that you need or want the abuser's approval. Trauma bonds get formed, in part, when you become addicted to this person's love, validation, and acceptance. Your partner has groomed you to need their approval. Ask yourself, though, why your partner, who is typically self-invested, would stay in a relationship with you if they genuinely believed you were "so terrible." Learning to question such illogicalness can help root out false guilt so that you can break free from abusive control. It is essential to recognize your bond with the abuser, though hard to break, is toxic, and the resulting guilt an illusion.

Self-Compassion

It is important to practice self-compassion and self-care. Be kind and gentle with yourself; remind yourself that you deserve to live in a safe and healthy environment.

Practicing self-compassion can be a powerful tool in healing. It is an effective way to overcome negative self-talk by recognizing that everyone is imperfect and makes mistakes. Show yourself the same measure of kindness and empathy that you would extend to someone else. A regular practice of self-compassion is an effective way to reduce stress and promote resilience. Here are some steps that can help:

1. Acknowledge negative self-talk: Become aware of your self-talk in a curious, non-judgmental way. Pay attention to the thoughts that come up when you're feeling guilty.

2. Challenge negative self-talk: Once you've identified it, challenge yourself by asking if it's true. Speak to yourself in the same thing you would talk to a friend. Question any harshness you feel toward yourself.

3. Reframe negative self-talk: Next, shift your negative self-talk statement(s) into something more positive and compassionate.

Here are two examples:

Negative self-talk: "I'm so stupid for staying with my abuser for so long."

Reframed self-talk: "It takes much courage to leave an abusive situation. I made the best decision I could then, and I'm proud of myself for taking steps towards healing."

Negative self-talk: "I'm a terrible person for letting my abuser hurt me."

Reframed self-talk: "I didn't deserve to be abused, and it's not my fault. I'm a strong person who's survived and am working on healing."

Reframing Negative Self-Talk

Acknowledge

Identify two negative things you've been telling yourself that is contributing to your guilt.

One:

_____

_____

Two:

_____

_____

Challenge

Is this true or false? List the evidence that supports this to be false.

One:

_____

_____

Two:

_____

_____

Reframe

Rewrite the beliefs into positive, compassionate statements.
One:

_____

_____

Two:

_____

_____

Self-Forgiveness

Focus on your own needs and priorities. Make self-care a priority, and pursue activities that bring you joy and fulfillment. It can be helpful to seek support from trusted friends, family members, or an informed coach or therapist who can provide emotional validation and help with perspective. Victims of abuse may have internalized messages from the abuser that they are to blame for the abuse.

Self-forgiveness is letting go of blame and guilt for past actions or decisions. Instead, move forward with self-compassion and understanding. Abuse victims often hold themselves responsible for getting into a toxic relationship or staying too long. Self-forgiveness also recognizes that no one deserves abuse, and those who harm us are solely responsible for their actions.

Practicing self-forgiveness reduces false guilt by acknowledging that we all are imperfect and capable of learning and growing from our mistakes.

Here are two ways to practice self-forgiveness:

- Write a letter to yourself: Take some time to reflect on the situation or decision causing guilt, and write a letter to yourself offering forgiveness and compassion. Acknowledge the painful difficulty of the circumstances, and remind yourself that you have done your best with the available information and resources.

- Practice self-compassion meditation: Set aside time to sit quietly and focus on your breath. Imagine breathing in love, compassion, and forgiveness as you inhale. As you exhale, imagine releasing feelings of guilt and self-blame. Repeat this process for several minutes, focusing on the warmth and kindness you extend toward yourself.

Sonni & McAvoy

Notes

Mastering Boundaries

Boundaries outline who we are. Just like our skin, they define us. They are the psychological, emotional, and physical perimeter of where another person ends and we begin. They encompass everything about us--our preferences, values, and beliefs. And they inform others what we are willing to accept and not accept when interacting with them, such as physical or emotional distance, communication styles, and respect levels.

Unfortunately, most of us have been socially conditioned to accept certain behaviors from others while neglecting our own needs. Boundary setting is especially problematic after abuse. Abusers condition us to think that their opinion is the absolute truth or that their needs should come first--definitely before ours.

Re-learning to set healthy personal limits is essential since it protects us from emotional and physical harm. Though not easy after living with an abuser who expected special treatment, it is a necessary part of healing after narcissistic abuse as we reclaim who we are and what's important to us.

Boundaries are not drawn to keep something out, but to protect what's in.

Unknown

MASTERING BOUNDARIES

Setting Boundaries

Setting boundaries is essential for maintaining healthy relationships. Boundaries are the limits we place on what we will and will not tolerate in our relationships with others. They are the guidelines we create to ensure that our needs are met, our values are respected, and our sense of self is protected. However, setting boundaries with a narcissistic or toxic person can be challenging.

Narcissists have a grandiose sense of self-importance, a need for admiration, and a lack of, or low, empathy. They see themselves as superior and expect others to treat them accordingly. Narcissists view boundaries as a personal challenge and often disregard or undermine them.

When attempting to set boundaries with a narcissist or toxic person, it is not uncommon for them to accuse you of trying to punish or control them. They may claim you are giving them ultimatums when you are simply asserting your right to be treated with respect and dignity. They often feel entitled to do as they please, regardless of how it impacts others, and view any attempt to limit their behavior as a personal attack. It is crucial to recognize that setting boundaries is not likely to change a narcissist's behavior. However, it can help protect you from further abuse.

It is important to remain calm, firm, and consistent when setting boundaries. Keep your expectations clear and communicate them in an assertive but not aggressive way. Avoid engaging in power struggles or arguments, as this will only fuel their need for control.

Remember, setting boundaries with a narcissist is not about changing them but protecting yourself. Be prepared to leave the relationship if they refuse to respect your limits. You always deserve to be treated with respect and dignity.

MASTERING BOUNDARIES

Your Beliefs About Boundaries

What beliefs have you held about boundaries? Do any of these sound familiar?

Saying "no" is selfish
I need to be liked by everyone
Setting boundaries will cause conflict
I should know what others need without them asking
My needs aren't as important as others' needs

People-pleasers often struggle with setting and holding boundaries because of a strong desire to keep others happy. As a result, they may have certain beliefs that make it difficult for them to establish and maintain healthy boundaries. Let's go through these.

1. Belief: "Saying 'no' is selfish." When saying 'no' to others is considered selfish, and the needs of others are prioritized over our own, we often become too agreeable and take on too much responsibility.

2. Belief: "I need to be liked by everyone." Placing a high value on being liked by others causes us to avoid setting boundaries out of fear of rejection. This tendency is heightened when we look to our partner for validation; anytime we attempt to place a limit, we face the possibility of rejection or abandonment.

3. Belief: "Setting boundaries will cause conflict." Since toxic people are antagonistic by nature, setting boundaries often leads to conflict or triggers the narcissist's rage, so we avoid enforcing limits to maintain peace.

4. Belief: "I should know what others need without them asking." Dysfunctional relationships often train us to anticipate others' needs and meet them without being asked.

5. Belief: "My needs aren't as important as others' needs." We place a lower priority on our needs and neglect setting boundaries to prioritize the needs of others.

It is crucial to recognize and challenge these beliefs if we want to get better at establishing healthy boundaries and prioritizing our needs.

Your Experience with Boundaries

What beliefs do you hold about boundaries?

_____

_____

_____

_____

What does/did your partner say about your boundaries?

_____

_____

_____

_____

How were you treated when you have attempted to set them?

_____

_____

_____

_____

Describe how boundaries were managed in your childhood home. Who set them and were they reasonable?

_____

_____

_____

_____

How did your parents respond to your preferences, likes/dislikes, and requests?

_____

_____

_____

Framework & Language

Boundaries provide the framework for communicating our needs and expectations in relationships. They protect us from people who do not always have our best interests at heart. Why is it so difficult to set our limitations? The answer lies in the purpose of boundaries. Behind each one is a value we hold dear—ourselves.

How Are Boundaries Different Than Threats or Ultimatums?

Here is an example: "If you disappear for long periods of time and I don't know where you are, then I am leaving you" vs. "I cannot be in a relationship where I cannot trust my partner." The first could be viewed as an ultimatum--based on fear and the need to control. The second is a request with clear boundaries.

Differences	Boundary	Ultimatium
Purpose	This is a personal limit that you establish to protect your physical, emotional, and mental well-being. It is a way of communicating to others what you are willing and unwilling to tolerate.	This is a demand that you make to someone else, with the intention of forcing them to change their behavior or actions.
Flexibility	It is flexible and adjustable over time as needs and circumstances change.	This is a rigid request with a "my way or the highway" mentality.
Control	This is something that you have control over, and is enforced with consequences when violated.	This is a demand of someone else, and compliance cannot be compelled.
Respect	This is an expression of your needs that demonstrates self-respect while honoring the boundaries of others.	This is experienced as disrespectful and can damage or destory relationships.

"You made me feel like crap when you said I am not a good cook. You always put me down." vs. "I felt hurt when you said I am not a good cook. I cannot be in a relationship where I am being insulted".

Statements that begin with "you" create defensiveness and feel like a personal attack. This is because they focus on the other person's behavior or actions. "You" statements come across as accusatory, critical, or judgmental, often conveying blame, shame, or disdain. Have you noticed how often a narcissistic or toxic person uses "you" statements? They put you on the defense, and victims usually respond as though attacked.

In contrast, "I" statements focus on the speaker's feelings and perceptions rather than the other person's behavior. These statements improve communication by reducing defensiveness and conveying empathy and understanding rather than blame and criticism. The second sentence in the above example is a boundary. It creates a framework of expectations of what you'll tolerate. Here is another example of an "I" statement: "I feel angry when I don't feel heard," which focuses on your feelings and perceptions rather than the other person's behavior.

Narcissistic or very toxic people don't generally respond well to either type of statement, but you have the best chance at success using "I" statements. It may be time to re-evaluate the relationship when and if these boundaries are still not respected.

4 Steps To Mastering Boundaries

1. Determine what is important and what boundaries need to be in place.
2. Evaluate the potential consequences if they are not respected.
3. Communicate your boundaries.
4. Follow through with consequences.

"Walls keep everybody out. Boundaries teach people where the door is.

Mark Groves

How To Set Boundaries

What Is Important

Core values are the guiding principles that shape your personality. They help you determine which people, goals, things, and decisions align with who you are. These principles influence your choices and decisions. While beliefs describe how you view the world, your actions demonstrate what matters to you. How you live out your core values will define you as an individual. Some examples of these are honesty, integrity, freedom, kindness, respect, forgiveness, and fairness.

Name three of your core values. How you are being treated or have been treated around each one?

_____

_____

_____

How does your life reflect or demonstrate each one of these values?

_____

_____

_____

What are some of the things that you believe are necessary for creating strong relationships?

_____

_____

_____

What are 3 boundaries you would like to set?

_____

_____

_____

How does the thought of setting these boundaries make you feel?

_____

_____

_____

Consider Consequences

Boundaries are only as effective as your ability to establish implementable consequences. You must assess your readiness to carry out any plan of action. You often know what you want to happen and what you are ready to make happen. Sometimes it is better to start with a lesser consequence until you are prepared to follow through on a greater one.

When setting limits with a narcissist, the consequences can be particularly significant since these individuals tend to disregard other people's boundaries. They prioritize their needs and desires above all else. Only set limits you can enforce. Any boundaries with unactionable consequences only weaken your position. You have signaled to narcissists that you lack the strength to hold your ground. This will result in further boundary violations, eroding your relationship's standing, self-worth, and autonomy. Examples of consequences for boundary violations may include limiting contact or ending the relationship altogether if they repeatedly refuse to respect your boundaries. Make sure that whatever consequence you establish, you can commit to. Communicate these outcomes clearly and calmly without engaging in arguments or becoming emotionally reactive.

What if you cannot end the relationship right now, or you're co-parenting and cannot go no contact? What consequences are you able to hold? Think of lesser, actionable limits, such as "I will end the call if there is any name-calling." The consequence could be that the conversation is over and that you will only reengage when the communication is calm and respectful.

List a consequence for each of the boundaries you've decided to set.

_____

_____

_____

Rate your preparedness to carry out each one on a scale of 1 to 10, with 10 being very ready.

1 - 2 - 3 - 4 - 5 - 6 - 7 - 8 - 9 - 10
not ready   very ready

Communicate Your Boundaries

Boundaries are difficult to enforce for several reasons. First, we may struggle to communicate our needs because we desire to please others. To secure love, validation, and acceptance from those around us, we may sacrifice caring for ourselves to gain their approval. This drive to please often is particularly challenging when dealing with a narcissist. Narcissists and other toxic people groom those around them to surrender their own needs and serve the narcissist instead. They use gaslighting and other forms of manipulation to convince us that our personal needs are unimportant or that boundary setting is selfish.

Secondly, those around us often encourage boundaries we are not ready to implement. Out of concern, our social support system may press for severe consequences, hoping these measures will protect us from further harm. This pressure may lead us to establish limits we cannot carry out, weakening our position with toxic people. We must listen to ourselves, particularly our readiness, when defining boundaries.

Thirdly, narcissistic, abusive, or toxic people are controlling. Healthy boundaries limit their power. Vested in avoiding external constraints, they often use persuasion, intimidation, or threats to convince us to remain passive and compliant. As a result, setting boundaries can feel scary.

Here are a few helpful tips when communicating boundaries:

- Use the J.A.D.E. method. Don't justify, argue, defend, or explain. State your limit firmly and dispassionately. Ignore any use of criticism or intimidation to confuse or control you.

- Be prepared for any possible reaction, and do not underestimate them. They have a lifetime of practicing manipulative strategies and are good at taking the upper hand.

- Be ready to be tested. They will try your resolve. Stand your ground. You may consider calling them out safely. If there is a risk of danger, have a plan of action in case of an emergency.

- Remember, how they respond does not matter. You are setting boundaries for yourself, not for them.

Consider the three new boundaries you would like to set and the level of preparedness you feel in holding them.

What factors are affecting your readiness?

_____

_____

_____

Are they realistic and enforceable? Why or why not?

_____

_____

_____

If not, what adjustment might be necessary to make them more doable?

_____

_____

_____

Based on past experiences, how do you anticipate your partner will react?

_____

_____

_____

How does your partner's possible response make you feel?

_____

_____

_____

What steps can you take to prepare yourself for this reaction?

_____

_____

_____

It is common to feel a need to overexplain new boundaries. That is not necessary. Remember, the purpose of limits is to show respect and care for yourself. It can be helpful to keep your statements short and to repeat them if necessary. Avoid defending yourself; simply hold your ground.

Here are some helpful phrases to consider if you experience any push-back, but remember that the most critical part is your execution of the consequence.

- "I understand that this may be uncomfortable for you, but it's necessary for me to have this boundary in order to feel safe and respected."

- "I understand that this may be difficult for you, but it's important for me to have this boundary in place."

- "I am not willing to compromise on this boundary, and it's not up for discussion."

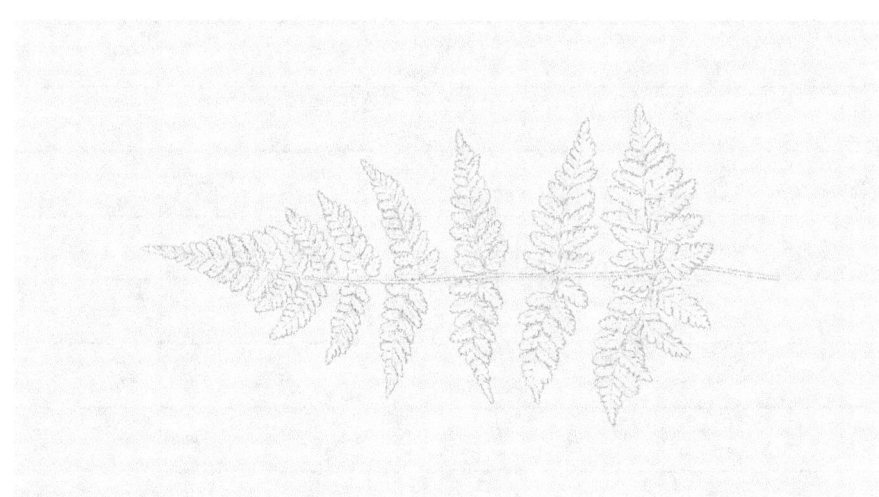

Notes

_____

_____

_____

_____

_____

_____

_____

_____

_____

_____

_____

_____

_____

_____

_____

_____

_____

_____

_____

_____

_____

_____

Developing Self-Worth

Experiencing abuse of any kind has a devastating impact on our self-worth. Narcissistic abuse, in particular, is uniquely damaging in its ability to chip away at our sense of self. The chronic experience of being manipulated, deceived, and betrayed begins to shape our self-perception.

We are born ready-made for healthy self-esteem. However, the process goes wrong when unresolved past experiences and emotions result in the development of negative beliefs about ourselves and the world around us. For instance, if someone important to us devalues or labels us as bad, we are at risk of unconsciously agreeing with them and experiencing ourselves the same way.

Knowing that this false perception has been a tool your abuser used for control can help you rebuild your self-worth from the ground up. Understanding this dynamic will help you dispel the lie and instead see yourself as someone who deserves respect, care, and concern.

Your self-worth doesn't belong in the hands of other people.

Ashley Hetherington

DEVELOPING SELF-WORTH

Self Worth vs. Self Esteem

Self-Worth: the internal sense of being good enough and worthy of love and belonging from others.

Self-Esteem: confidence in one's own worth or abilities

Self-esteem relies on external factors such as successes and achievements to define value, which can be inconsistent, leading to internal struggles of unworthiness. Self-esteem is the appraisal of one's self-worth.

Low self-worth occurs when individuals have an overall negative opinion of themselves and is characterized by self-criticism, self-doubt, and an inability to recognize positive personal qualities. People with low self-worth often view themselves negatively, leading to feelings of unworthiness, inferiority, and a lack of confidence. It is based on inaccurate and distorted self-perceptions. Individuals with low self-worth often hold themselves to unrealistic standards and compare themselves unfavorably to others. This problem occurs when an internalized pattern of self-deprecation and insecurity develops from receiving long-standing negative feedback.

Define how you view yourself.

_____

_____

_____

Where is this self-perception derived from?

_____

_____

_____

How do I think, feel, and act because of this assessment?

_____

_____

_____

Sonni & McAvoy

DEVELOPING SELF-WORTH

The Roots of Self-Worth

Let's go back to infancy to explore how the sense of self is developed.

Our initial experience of care forms our earliest perceptions of ourselves and our worth--a safe and secure home life builds trust. The warmth & safety found in the caregiver's arms create good feelings. Unconsciously the baby concludes from "this is pleasing" to "I have value." This process is reinforced when the child feels cherished, understood, and praised. As a result, the growing self becomes confident with high self-esteem. This psychological connection between care and self-perception becomes the foundation for future self-definition.

The opposite happens in chaotic, overly rigid, or critical homes. These children equate a childhood home of insecurity with "I must be bad or unworthy." Unfair or excessive punishment and criticism can further erode the child's vulnerable sense of self.

This process does not stop in adulthood. Throughout life, the sense of self or "ego" continues to be influenced by shifting family roles, social interactions, and life experiences. Outside influences impact self-perception, such as social acceptance or rejection, and positive or negative experiences, such as bullying and abuse. Unresolved past experiences and emotions can lead to negative beliefs about ourselves and the world, perpetuating a cycle of self-doubt and low self-esteem.

Every moment either builds or erodes our sense of self.

Here are some things that can negatively impact our self-concept:

- Neglectful or abusive homes
- Unpredictable or unstable home life
- early loss, an alcoholic parent, parents' divorce, overly chaotic or rigid
- Neglectful or overly-involved caregivers
- A poor connection with parents or care providers
- Excessive criticism or control
- Stressful or traumatic life events
- Chronic illness of a parent or sibling

The History of Your Self-Development

Our first experiences are critical in the development of our self-concept. During these formative years, our brains rapidly acquire new skills, such as motor coordination, oral and written language, imagination, and the earliest beginnings of socialization. Our caregivers' reactions either encouraged our crude efforts or made us hesitant and fearful, leaving us feeling confident or ashamed.

Think back to your earliest memories of home. How would you describe that environment? Playful, structured, predictable, chaotic, warm, encouraging, scary, etc.?

How do you remember feeling in your home?

_____

_____

_____

Who was safe and why?

_____

_____

_____

Who was unsafe and why?

_____

_____

_____

Our sense of self continues to evolve in adulthood, although less dramatically. Our personal accomplishments and outside relationships influence how we see ourselves. Outside experiences, such as school, extracurricular activities, and among our peers, are incorporated into our evolving self-concept, confirming or invalidating earlier self-definitions.

Which outside experiences impacted you?

_____

_____

_____

Describe how these affected your self-perception.

_____

_____

_____

As we mature, we build a catalog of life successes and failures and a belief system about what they mean. Adult relationships become the primary sources for our still malleable self-perception but to a lesser degree than the ones we had with our parents. Now other life experiences play an essential role in how we see ourselves, such as our work life and personal accomplishments. Even our self-care shapes our internal sense of having value.

Define how you viewed yourself as a young adult.

_____

_____

_____

Describe which early adulthood experiences or relationships played a vital role in that definition.

_____

_____

_____

Abusive relationships, particularly narcissistic abuse, dramatically affect our self-concept. Narcissists and toxic partners use a system of psychological rewards and punishments to gain compliance. Gaslighting, lying, and misdirection distort reality and confuse the victim. To maintain control, narcissists use criticism, emotional withholding, and deprivation to keep their partners off-balanced and vulnerable. All of this causes victims to question themselves and their experience of reality. Cognitive dissonance leads to a deterioration of mental functioning, making victims less confident, while the abuse erodes their self-perception.

Describe at least three tactics your current or ex-partner kept you confused and off-balance.

_____

_____

_____

Affirmation and Mindsets

Affirmations can powerfully shift our mindset and help us develop a more positive self-image. However, repeating positive statements without evidence or buy-in can sometimes feel disingenuous or even counterproductive. It's essential to tap into our own experiences and beliefs to create affirmations that truly resonate.

"What evidence do I have to support my affirmations?"

Rather than repeating general positive statements, remember when you demonstrated the qualities or traits you want to embody and use those experiences to create positive affirmations.

For example, instead of saying, "I am confident," you might say, "I have overcome challenges in the past and can handle whatever comes my way with confidence and grace."

"What areas of my life do I want to focus on?"

Think of the areas you want to improve, such as relationships, career, health, or personal development. Consider brainstorming motivating or inspiring statements that address those specific arenas and use those to create relevant and meaningful affirmations.

For example, to focus on improving relationships, you might create affirmations like "I am a good listener and communicator" or "I show up for my loved ones with love and compassion."

"What kind of care and support am I worthy of because I exist?"

Finally, consider the encouragement and support we deserve because of our humanity. These are things we freely give to our children and loved ones. It's important we also invest in ourselves in the same ways.

For example, to improve your sense of value and self-worth, you might create affirmations like "I am worthy of love and support" or "It's okay when I make mistakes because failure is a part of learning."

Sonni & McAvoy

Putting New Beliefs into Practice

Define your current self-beliefs.

_____

_____

_____

_____

_____

Are these reasonable, helpful, or positive?

_____

_____

_____

_____

Why or why not?

_____

_____

_____

Write a negative one that is currently having the most impact on you.

_____

_____

_____

_____

Identify a few reasons why this belief is not valid, unreasonable, or unfair.

_____

_____

_____

_____

_____

Based on past experiences and what you know to be true, create a new one to replace it.

_____

_____

_____

_____

_____

The next time you catch yourself stating this negative statement, replace it with the new one. At first, this will feel awkward. Push through those feelings and repeat the new affirmation as often as you need; over time, it will begin to feel real.

Notes

_____

_____

_____

_____

_____

_____

_____

_____

_____

_____

_____

_____

_____

_____

_____

_____

_____

_____

_____

_____

_____

Closing

As we reach the end of *Surviving To Thriving: A Six-Step Blueprint to Narcissistic Abuse Recovery and Healing*, we want to acknowledge the tremendous courage and resilience you have displayed throughout this journey. It is our hope that the insights, activities, and tools within these pages have provided you with the support and guidance necessary to overcome the obstacles you have faced and have set you on a path towards healing and self-discovery. The journey to recovery from narcissistic abuse is not linear; there may be times when you feel the need to revisit certain sections of this workbook. Please remember that this is completely normal. Healing takes time, patience, and self-compassion.

From our hearts to yours, we want to express our deepest gratitude for allowing us to be a part of your healing journey. We are honored to have walked this path with you and to have witnessed the your incredible show of strength and resilience. As you continue to grow and thrive, know that you are never alone. And never forget that you hold the power to create a life full of joy and fulfillment.

With warmth and gratitude

Lisa & Kerry

Lisa Sonni & Kerry Kerr McAvoy, PhD

Follow the Authors

Lisa Sonni

Website: https://strongerthanbefore.ca

SOCIAL MEDIA
Instagram: @_stronger_than_before_coaching
YouTube: @strongerthanbefore
TikTok: @_stronger_than_before_

Kerry Kerr McAvoy, Ph. D.

Website: https://kerrymcavoyphd.com

SOCIAL MEDIA
Instagram: @kerrymcavoyphd
YouTube: @kerrymcavoyphd
TikTok: @kerrymcavoyphd
Podcast: Breaking Free from Narcissistic Abuse

www.ingramcontent.com/pod-product-compliance
Lightning Source LLC
Chambersburg PA
CBHW071213120626
46546CB00006B/2544